Published in association with

THE BRITISH
DIGESTIVE
FOUNDATION

BRITISH DIGESTIVE FOUNDATION

Telling the Inside Story

The British Digestive Foundation (BDF) was set up
in 1971 by gastroenterologists to:

Fund new research into digestive diseases
Provide information to the public
Offer sufferers practical guidelines

The BDF raises funds to provide research training fellowships to
encourage those with academic promise. The BDF also aims to
prevent people from suffering in silence: the "All About" leaflets
provide clear, general information for lay people on common
digestive disorders, while the "Understanding" booklets - for health
professionals to give to patients - give a deeper insight into certain
conditions.

Donations to, and further information from:
British Digestive Foundation, 3 St Andrew's Place, London NW1 4LB

GASTROCARE

DIAGNOSIS & MANAGEMENT THROUGH SYMPTOMS

Dyspepsia

I Finnie
Glan Clwyd Hospital
North Wales, UK

DE Loft
Walsgrave Hospital
Coventry, UK

MJG Farthing (Series Editor)
St Bartholomew's Hospital
London, UK

SCIENCE PRESS

British Library Cataloguing-in-Publication Data
A catalogue record for this book is available from the British Library.

ISBN: 1-85873-005-8

This copy of *Gastrocare: Dyspepsia* is given as a service to medicine by Lederle Laboratories. Sponsorship of this copy does not imply the sponsor's agreement or otherwise with the views expressed herein.

Although every effort has been made to ensure that drug doses and other information are presented accurately in this publication, the ultimate responsibility rests with the prescribing physician. Neither the publishers nor the authors can be held responsible for errors or for any consequences arising from the use of the information contained herein. Any product mentioned in this publication should be used in accordance with the prescribing information prepared by the manufacturers. No claims or endorsements are made for any drug or compound at present under clinical investigation.

Project editors: Sara Churchill and Alison Taylor
Illustrator: Daniel Simmons
Typesetter: Paul Angliss
Production: Rebecca Spencer
Printed in Wales by Pensord Press

Preface

Our understanding of the causes and management of dyspepsia has changed dramatically during the past two decades. When I was a medical student (not so long ago!) the standard therapy for a peptic ulcer was an antacid, possibly combined with carbenoxolone. As a registrar I was involved in the early studies with H_2-receptor antagonists, which many of us believed at the time were going to be unsurpassable remedies for the treatment of ulceration and reflux. Two major developments, however, soon followed, namely the discovery of *Helicobacter pylori* and the characterization of the proton pump with the development of drugs to inhibit its action. Thus, the aetiopathogenesis of peptic ulceration has been turned on its head, and new powerful agents have emerged for acid inhibition and the treatment of acid related disorders. Is this the end to the story? What can we expect to see in the future?

These are interesting times in which new ideas about the mechanisms and management of gastrointestinal disorders continue to evolve. This book on 'dyspepsia' is one of a series aimed at presenting current views on the management of common clinical problems in gastroenterology. In this volume the authors have dealt with some of the controversial issues in diagnosis and management of dyspepsia in a careful and succinct manner. Our aim has been to produce a readable and clinically useful text which, at least for 1994, is state-of-the-art. No doubt the story will continue to evolve, our ideas will change and new recommendations emerge.

MJG Farthing
April 1994

Author biographies

Professor Michael Farthing is Professor of Gastroenterology, St Bartholomew's Hospital, London. He graduated from University College, London and University College Hospital and held positions in London and Cambridge. Professor Farthing was a Research Fellow at St Mark's Hospital and St Bartholomew's Hospital where he completed his doctoral research and clinical training. He spent two years at Tufts University School of Medicine, Boston, in the Department of Geographic Medicine and returned to St Bartholomew's Hospital in 1983 as a Wellcome Senior Lecturer. He became Professor of Gastroenterology at St Bartholomew's Hospital Medical College in 1990. He serves on a number of editorial boards and is currently Secretary of the British Society of Gastroenterology, Director of the Post Graduate Medical Foundation Advanced Course in Gastroenterology and an active supporter of the British Digestive Foundation and the National Association for Colitis and Crohns' Disease.

Dr Ian Finnie has recently been appointed Consultant Physician and Gastroenterologist at Glan Clwyd Hospital, North Wales. He graduated from Aberdeen University and held clinical positions in Aberdeen and Merseyside. He was a Reseach Fellow in the University of Liverpool and did much of his clinical training at the Royal Liverpool University Hospital. His publications include original articles on the aetiology of inflammatory bowel disease, therapeutic endoscopy and colonic mucin synthesis. Dr Finnie's current clinical and research interests include inflammatory bowel disease, endoscopy and intestinal permeability.

Dr Duncan Loft is Consultant Physician and Gastroenterologist at the Walsgrave Hospital NHS Trust, Coventry, UK. After a three year period of basic science doctoral research as MRC Research Fellow at Hope Hospital, Manchester, he completed his higher medical training as Senior Registrar at the Central Middlesex Hospital and St Mary's Hospital, London. His clinical and research interests include peptic ulcer disease, oesophageal carcinoma, all aspects of therapeutic endoscopy and ERCP, *Helicobacter pylori*, cellular immunology and coeliac disease. He acts as invited refereee for several gastroenterological journals and is co-editor of "Current Medical Literature — Gastroenterology" (Royal Society of Medicine).

Contents

Introduction

Dyspepsia is a symptom complex which may include epigastric pain, heartburn or nausea and sometimes upper abdominal bloating. The scale of the symptom complex poses a massive problem: 25% of the UK population are affected by dyspepsia at some time and the symptoms account for 4% of all general practice consultations. Clearly, not all these patients need to be investigated; most can be treated empirically without further investigation. Many clinicians worry about missing serious underlying disease, including malignancy, but careful diagnosis and rational treatment as outlined on the following pages should alleviate this worry.

The last 20 years have seen a swing from surgical to medical management of peptic ulcer and gastro-oesophageal reflux disease (GORD). The introduction of more potent acid inhibitors has offered symptom relief and healing of the most resistant cases of GORD. Knowledge of the underlying mechanisms of peptic ulcer disease (for example, the on-going elucidation of the role of *Helicobacter pylori*) has increased dramatically, leading to new treatment strategies such as the use of anti-microbial therapy in combination with acid suppression.

This handbook provides a rationale for deciding which patients with dyspepsia should be investigated and how they should be managed.

I Finnie
DE Loft

1 Diagnosis

1.1 PRESENTATION AND HISTORY TAKING

Characteristically, the patient with dyspepsia presents with epigastric pain or retrosternal burning. Together with nausea, flatulence, vomiting, post-prandial fullness, bloating and regurgitation, these features make up the symptom complex known as dyspepsia. The aim of taking a history is to:

1. Establish the presence or absence of classic symptoms from which a clinical diagnosis may be made;

2. Exclude sinister symptoms, which will require further investigation, before trials of symptomatic treatment;

3. Identify atypical symptoms that might suggest a condition other than one traditionally associated with dyspepsia.

Patients with upper gastrointestinal symptoms pose a major diagnostic problem to the clinician. Even the most experienced doctor can only expect to predict the correct diagnosis in 45–50% of cases [1.1]. Accuracy can be improved by the use of a structured questionnaire, but this approach is cumbersome and has never gained widespread acceptability. Recognizing specific symptom patterns can help the practitioner arrive at the correct diagnosis.

Clues from the history
Pain
Most patients will complain of pain or discomfort to a greater or lesser extent, but may have difficulty describing it. The essential features to elicit are shown on page 2. The **site**, **radiation** and **referral** of pain should be confirmed by examining the patient because seated patients sometimes indicate a site of pain remote from the area where the pain is actually felt.

Pain which radiates to the back may be suggestive of biliary or pancreatic disease.

Essential features of abdominal pain
• Site
• Radiation and referral
• Character
• Timing
• Modifying features
• Associated symptoms
• Psychological background

Radiation to the shoulder tip is usually considered to represent diaphragmatic irritation but is also found in the 'splenic flexure' variant of irritable bowel syndrome. The **character of pain** is probably the most difficult aspect for the patient to describe, but an accurate description can be useful. Certain conditions produce pain with characteristic qualities, for example:

• Peptic ulcer is associated with a gnawing epigastric discomfort.

• Biliary pain is severe and short-lived, and well remembered by the patient.

• Gastro-oesophageal reflux disease (GORD) is associated with a burning sensation in the chest.

Description of the **timing of pain** should include the **frequency** and **duration** of intermittent symptoms, the **time of day** at which the symptoms occur, as well as the **long-term pattern** of pain.

• The epigastric pain of peptic ulcer is typically thought of as occurring at night, with periods of several days or weeks free from symptoms between episodes of pain.

• Biliary pain is typically severe, constant in intensity and occurs in sudden episodes which are unpredictable.

Pain which wakes the patient from sleep is typical of organic disease. Modifying features are particularly helpful in the diagnosis. Specific enquiry should be made about the relationship of symptoms to **meals, hunger, posture** and **exercise** and **self medication with antacids**.

• Most patients will volunteer the relationship between their symptoms and spicy foods, but there is no good evidence that exacerbation of symptoms with such food is discriminatory for peptic ulcer. The same can be said for the erroneous association between gallstone disease symptoms induced by fatty food. Food intolerance is common; allergy is extremely rare.

• The relationship to meals, irrespective of their content, is of more help. For example, symptoms which occur on an empty stomach and are relieved by food are characteristic of duodenal ulcer.

- Epigastric or chest pain which is exacerbated on lying down is highly suggestive of GORD.

- The relief of pain with antacids does not necessarily discriminate peptic ulcer disease from other diseases [1.2].

Symptoms associated with the pain, such as **bloating** and **belching**, can be diagnostically useful. For example, bloating or belching in the absence of any abnormality on examination, are suggestive of a functional disturbance with aerophagy. Vomiting and weight loss are suggestive of organic disease.

In the absence of any identifiable organic disease the patient's **psychological background** may be relevant. Approximately half of all patients with symptoms associated with the upper gastrointestinal tract referred to hospital are found to have an organic disease [1.2]. The definition and classification of this group is made easier by the use of objective criteria which are universally agreed.

The remaining patients do not have identifiable organic disease, and are usually said to suffer from functional dyspepsia, nervous dyspepsia or non-ulcer dyspepsia. Classification of this group of patients is much more difficult because of the lack of formal criteria for diagnosis. It is often, but not always, possible to make a positive diagnosis on the basis of a good clinical history. Emotional or psychiatric disturbance is almost always denied at first, but careful establishment of rapport may lead to the patient admitting lack of drive or energy, poor concentration and memory, tiredness or apathy, all of which suggest depression. Patients may have a long history of somatic symptoms, such as headache or low backache, suggestive of other disease but for which no organic cause was ever found.

Heartburn

If heartburn and acid regurgitation are prominent features, gastro-oesophageal reflux is frequently found.

Atypical presentations

The problem of the occurrence of symptoms in the absence of organic disease has already been discussed. The opposite scenario can be considered to be patients with chest or epigastric pain who on thorough investigation are found to have more than one potential explanation for their symptoms. Indeed, of all patients with symptoms of upper gastrointestinal disease in whom an organic cause for is found, 25% are shown to have more than one organic disease to explain them. It is possible that some people are truly symptomatic from separate conditions, but it is clear from investigation of asymptomatic individuals that gallstones and apparently significant peptic ulceration can exist in the absence of symptoms. Thus, when patients with atypical symp-

Typical features of specific diseases of the upper gastrointestinal tract	
Duodenal ulcer	**Gastro-oesophageal reflux disease**
Frequent nocturnal epigastric pain	Chest/epigastric pain on bending/stooping/lying down
Relief with food/milk	Reflux of food/acid into throat and mouth
Chronic pain for weeks interspersed by weeks without pain	Associated use of tobacco and alcohol
Associated use of tobacco/excess alcohol	
Family history, pointing sign, long history (> 4 yrs)	
Gall bladder/biliary tract disease	**Gastric ulcer**
Episodic severe pain but constant for duration of episode	More common if aged between 41–55 yrs
No pain on an empty stomach	Pain exacerbated by food
Pain may radiate to back	
Pale stools, dark urine, jaundice, fever or rigors, abnormal liver enzymes — all suggestive of bile duct calculi	
Gastric cancer	**Functional abdominal pain**
More common if age > 55 yrs	More common in young women
Daily pain	Prominent bloating/belching
Vomiting of dark fluid	Previous somatic symptoms, e.g. headache, low backache
Weight loss	Tiredness, lack of drive
Early satiety	Associated symptoms of altered bowel habit
History > 1 yr	
The presence of these features is suggestive of the diagnosis but their absence does not necessarily indicate that this diagnosis is incorrect	

toms are found to have a peptic ulcer, whether the symptoms relate to the ulcer can only be a matter of conjecture. In such a situation, ulcer-healing (confirmed endoscopically) with resolution of symptoms, would help suggest whether the symptoms and ulcer were connected.

Sinister symptoms

The greatest risk of inaccurate or delayed diagnosis is missing a patient with malignant disease. The demographic features of malignant disease are such that malignancy is very unlikely to cause epigastric pain or heartburn in the absence of sinister symptoms in patients under the age of 45 years. Dysphagia (difficulty swallowing) and odynophagia (pain on swallowing) occurring in a patient *de novo* are usually an indicator of organic oesophageal disease and should prompt further and urgent investigation. Statistically more men have a malignant cause for these symptoms, largely because functional abdominal pain occurs more frequently in women. Sinister symptoms that justify investigation for cancer include: weight loss, vomiting dark fluid/haematemesis, melaena, anorexia, dysphagia, odynophagia and constant daily pain.

1.2 PHYSICAL EXAMINATION

1. The patient's weight should be recorded and compared with previous measurements.

2. General inspection may reveal evidence of anaemia, jaundice, tar-stained fingers, cachexia, supraclavicular or generalized lymphadenopathy (benign peptic ulcer disease does not cause chronic iron-deficiency anaemia; another cause of the anaemia should be sought).

3. Abdominal examination is the most important part of a physical examination for upper gastrointestinal tract disease. Epigastric tenderness is suggestive of peptic ulceration; a mass may suggest pancreatic or other malignancy. The presence of any mass, its size, consistency, and relationship to respiration should be noted. In patients who have prominent bloating and/or vomiting, remember to examine for the presence of a succussion splash.

4. Rectal examination is mandatory and may reveal melaena.

Physical examination of a patient with gastro-oesophageal reflux, uncomplicated peptic ulcer, gallstones, or pancreatic disease will often reveal no abnormality.

Important considerations in the diagnosis of upper gastrointestinal tract disease
• Age — in the absence of sinister symptoms an underlying malignancy is unlikely under the age of 45 years
• Past medical history — may reveal previous peptic ulcer surgery
• Medication — in particular, enquire about the use of NSAIDS
• Social history — smoking retards ulcer healing and increases the likelihood of relapse. Alcohol relaxes the lower oesophageal sphincter and may aggravate GORD. Certain occupations may aggravate GORD particularly if stooping is involved, e.g. carpet fitting
• Family history — first-degree relatives of patients with duodenal ulceration are affected in about 20% of cases, compared with an overall 10% prevalence in the UK

1.3 PRELIMINARY AND DIFFERENTIAL DIAGNOSIS

After taking a thorough history and performing a clinical examination, it should be possible to make a provisional diagnosis. This will not always be confirmed by further investigation, and it is by no means unusual for the investigations to reveal an abnormality which was thought unlikely from the preceding history and examination.

Differential diagnosis of patients presenting with dyspepsia
Variants of peptic ulcer disease
Presents with characteristic symptoms of peptic ulcer disease (see p4)
• Gastro-oesophageal reflux disease
• Gastric ulcer
• Duodenal ulcer
• Non-ulcer dyspepsia including gastritis and duodenitis

Differential diagnosis of patients presenting with dyspepsia (continued)
Variants of non-peptic ulcer disease
May present with sinister symptoms (see p5)

- Oesophageal or gastric cancer
- Non-peptic inflammation including: Crohn's disease, HIV-related infections, cytomegalovirus infection
- Gallstone disease
- Pancreatic disease
- Angina
- Colonic pathology
- Irritable bowel syndrome

Differential diagnosis — atypical presentation
Some patients with peptic ulcer present with atypical symptoms, e.g.:

- Chest pain presenting erroneously as angina
- Right upper quadrant pain presenting erroneously as gall-stone disease
- Back pain presenting erroneously as pancreatic disease

1.4 INVESTIGATIONS

Many investigations can be considered to confirm a diagnosis in a patient with dyspepsia. The relative merits of these investigations are discussed here.

Routine biochemical/haematological tests

- A full blood count can reveal anaemia, suggest iron deficiency or, more rarely, thrombocytosis, if there has been recurrent bleeding. In the absence of overt bleeding anaemia is not caused by a simple peptic ulcer and another explanation should be sought.

- Elevated erythrocyte sedimentation rate (ESR) might suggest Crohn's disease or vasculitis.

- Serum electrolytes might reveal evidence of renal failure, hypercalcaemia or, in unusual cases, suggest Addison's disease.

Endoscopy

In the last 15–20 years the management of patients with dyspepsia has been revolutionized by the widespread availability of endoscopy. There has been considerable debate about whether this is beneficial to patients, doctors or health care budgets. The value of a specific investigation is very difficult to prove, but audits on the usefulness or cost-benefit of endoscopy are becoming more numerous and should help to clarify the situation. Complication rates from peptic ulcer have remained static in the last 20 years, suggesting that the prevalence of the disease is probably unchanged, but that the number of endoscopies has risen

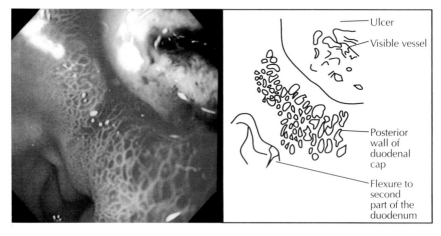

Endoscopic photograph of duodenal cap containing a large posterior wall duodenal ulcer. The patient has presented with haematemesis and malaena. There is a vessel at the base of the ulcer which has recently bled.

Endoscopy	
Advantages	**Disadvantages**
• Good for diagnosis of mucosal abnormalities	• Some associated morbidity (small)
• Lesions can be biopsied to assess malignancy or otherwise	• Some associated mortality (very small)
• Allows therapeutic procedures, e.g. dilation of strictures, relieving malignant obstruction	• Not sensitive for assessing anatomy or gastro-oesophageal reflux

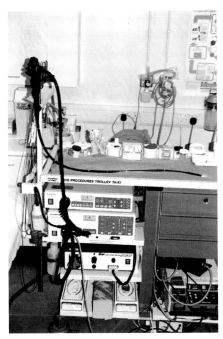

steadily. There is good evidence, however, that endoscopy should be regarded as the gold standard for investigation of mucosal ulceration, although attaching undue importance to minor erosions and gastritis is a common problem. Endoscopy of asymptomatic people reveals one or more minor abnormalities in over half, and difficulty may arise in interpreting whether the symptoms and the endoscopic abnormality are related.

Open-access endoscopy implies that the decision to proceed with the investigation is taken by the general practitioner, in much the same way that barium meal examinations have been ordered by general practitioners for many years. This is a relatively recent development which has not gained universal approval. The main arguments for the open-access

Standard endoscopic equipment prior to use.

system are economic; the time and money saved by not reviewing such patients in clinic first can theoretically be used for other purposes. Those who are against open-access endoscopy state that all patients with symptoms bad

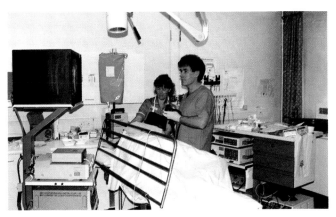

A modern purpose-built endoscopy unit.

9

Patient information: endoscopy

- Usually done as an out-patient procedure, ideally in a purpose-built endoscopy suite

- The procedure will be explained and a consent form presented to the patient for signature

- The examination is short, 5–10 minutes unless a biopsy has to be taken or a treatment procedure is required

- Before starting, the oropharynx is sometimes sprayed with a local anaesthetic. In many cases an intravenous sedative will also be given

- The endoscope is fed through the mouth, pharynx and oesophagus into the stomach and duodenum

- A report on the results should be sent to the general practitioner the same day (most units now have computerized records which will allow quick dispatch)

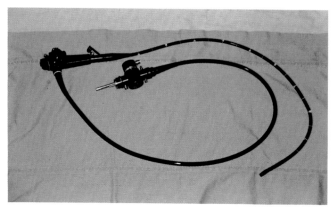

Photograph of a video oesophago-gastroduodeno-scope. A selection of endoscopes with different characteristics are available for various diagnostic and therapeutic applications.

enough to warrant endoscopy should merit review by a specialist in the field. In practice, most hospitals already have sizeable waiting lists for endoscopy and may not be adequately resourced to take on what is generally perceived to be an increased workload.

Barium meal

The increasing use of endoscopy has been mirrored by a decrease in the number of barium meal examinations. It is generally accepted that endoscopy is the more sensitive technique; approximately 10% of ulcers that are seen at endoscopy are missed by barium meal examination (although very few clinically significant or sinister lesions will be missed by this technique). Inevitably, because of the length of the waiting time for endoscopy, some patients are sent first for a barium examination. If an abnormality, which then requires biopsy, is revealed by barium studies or if the test is normal and symptoms continue, then endoscopy might be required.

Patient information: barium meal
• Usually done as an outpatient procedure
• Requires the patient to take no food or drink four hours before the test
• Non-invasive, causes minimal discomfort, if any, but involves radiation

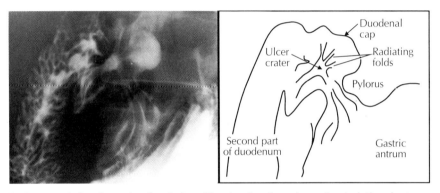

Barium meal showing a duodenal ulcer. The duodenal cap is contracted; the ulcer crater and radiating folds can be seen.

Barium meal	
Advantages	**Disadvantages**
• Good for assessing anatomy, e.g. presence of strictures, hiatus hernia	• Interpretation can be difficult in patients who have had previous gastric surgery
• Often more readily available than endoscopy	• Less sensitive than endoscopy in assessing mucosal lesions
• Can be used to observe reflux episodes	• Cumulative radiation risk if a large dose is repeatedly used

Oesophageal pH monitoring

This is the most sensitive and specific investigation for the diagnosis of GORD. Although it is usually organised by specialist centres, monitoring is normally done on an out-patient basis to allow correlation of the patient's symptoms with their normal activity, for example, meals or stooping down. It also allows

---

Patient information: oesophageal pH monitoring

• This test measures the acidity of the oesophagus over time

• A narrow tube called a pH probe is inserted through the nose into the oesophagus and is usually left in place for 24 hours

• The probe is connected to a recorder (worn in a holster like a large Walkman holder)

• Normal activities (eating, sleeping, etc.) should be maintained while the probe is in place — the machine will carry on recording

• When an attack of 'burning' pain comes on, the manual marker should be activated. Later, this will enable the consultant to correlate symptoms with oesophageal pH

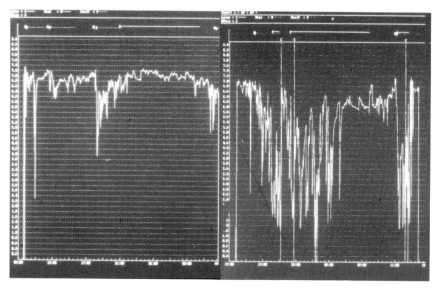

Oesophageal pH monitoring. Trace showing normal pH change (left) and abnormal pH change (right); event markers such as meals and chest pain (c) are recorded with the use of a manual marker. Published by permission of JS de Caestecker, Glenfield Hospital, Leicester, UK.

Oesophageal pH monitoring	
Advantages	**Disadvantages**
• Can be done as an out-patient procedure	• Limited direct access for general practitioners
• Diagnostic for gastro-oesophageal reflux if pH < 4 for more than 4% of 24-hour period	• Impact on patient's lifestyle for period of monitoring
• Allows quantitation of acid reflux	• Requires patient compliance for accurate recording

a quantative assessment of the degree of acid reflux, and a direct correlation between the patients symptoms and the reflux episodes. In the normal individual, oesophageal pH should not fall below 4 for more than 4% of a 24 hour period.

Other investigations
Oesophageal manometry
• Used to measure motility, peristalsis and lower oesophageal sphincter relaxation
• Not usually appropriate for patients presenting with dyspepsia except in the investigation of atypical non-cardiac chest pain or dysphagia
Upper abdominal ultrasound
• Procedure of choice for the diagnosis of gallstones but may miss stones in the common bile duct
• Almost as sensitive as computerized tomography for imaging the pancreas
• Readily available, often on open access
• No associated morbidity
Computerized tomography
• Procedure of choice for diagnosis of pancreatic lesions
• Requires significant radiation dose
• Limited availability

1.5 WHETHER TO REFER

The decision to refer a patient for endoscopy and/or further investigation must ultimately rest with the general practitioner, and research shows that practitioners vary greatly in their referral rates. Some general advice, however, can be given which is summarized as follows.

Criteria for referral
Refer if:
• Sinister symptoms are present (see p5)
• The patient is over 45 years of age and has typical symptoms which recur after one month of treatment
• Complications of peptic ulcer occur, e.g. pyloric stenosis, haemorrhage
• The patient has a known gastric ulcer
• Symptoms recur from a previously known gastric ulcer
• Anxiety about the diagnosis exists in either the patient or GP
Think twice about referring if:
• Patient has a known duodenal ulcer from a previous presentation
• No treatment with antacid or acid-suppressing medication has been attempted *and*
• Symptoms are typical
• Patient is under 45 years of age
• First presentation with symptoms

1.6 IS MAKING A SPECIFIC DIAGNOSIS NECESSARY?

To investigate all patients at their first presentation with dyspepsia is impractical. The clinician may worry about missing a tumour but this is unlikely if the patient has typical symptoms, is under 45 years of age, it is the initial presentation, there has been no trial of antacid or acid-suppressing medication or if the patient has a history of known duodenal ulcer disease.

Furthermore, in the first instance, an accurate diagnosis may not be necessary. If the patient has characteristic symptoms of dyspepsia then a course of treatment with an antisecretory agent is justified. The proton-pump inhibitors (see pp20–21) are such powerful acid-suppressing agents that if a patient's symptoms do not abate after two weeks of treatment (e.g. lansoprazole 30 mg or omeprazole 20 mg once daily), the symptoms are unlikely to be acid-related.

It is not necessary to know the *Helicobacter pylori* status of the patient unless the case is one of recurrent duodenal ulcer which requires triple therapy (see pp25–26). Endoscopy is not performed merely to assess the *H. pylori* status.

A specific diagnosis is necessary if:

- Sinister symptoms are present (see p5).
- The patient is aged over 45 years and has characteristic symptoms which recur after one month of treatment.
- There are complications of peptic ulceration.
- There is a known gastric ulcer.
- There are recurrent symptoms from previously established gastric ulcer.
- There is anxiety about the working diagnosis from either the patient or general practitioner.

1.7 SUMMARY

- A good history and thorough clinical examination are vital aspects of management.
- If the history is characteristic of duodenal ulcer, gastro-oesophageal reflux, or a non-organic cause, treat accordingly (see pp19–26).
- Patients with persistent or sinister symptoms, particularly older patients (age over 45 years), should be investigated early.
- The free availability of endoscopy is not a substitute for taking a good history.
- Symptoms are not a good indicator of the severity of disease.

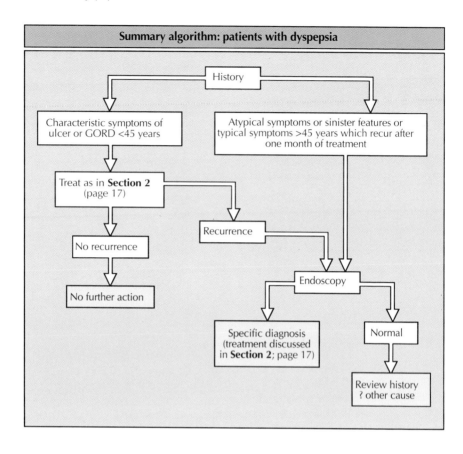

Summary algorithm: patients with dyspepsia

History

Characteristic symptoms of ulcer or GORD <45 years

Atypical symptoms or sinister features or typical symptoms >45 years which recur after one month of treatment

Treat as in **Section 2** (page 17)

No recurrence

Recurrence

No further action

Endoscopy

Specific diagnosis (treatment discussed in **Section 2**; page 17)

Normal

Review history ? other cause

2 Treatment

2.1. PRINCIPAL DRUGS FOR THE TREATMENT OF PEPTIC ULCERATION AND GASTRO-OESOPHAGEAL REFLUX DISEASE

Summary of principal drugs for peptic ulceration and gastro-oesophageal reflux disease			
Drug	Dose	*Cost	Comment
Antacids/ alignates	5–20 ml or 1 tab. ≥ four times daily	£1.50– £10.00	Side effects include constipation (aluminium), diarrhoea (magnesium); some contain large amounts of Na^+ and so care must be taken in patients with heart failure
H-2-receptor antagonists			
Cimetidine	400 mg twice daily or 800 mg at night	£10.00– £20.00	Interactions with oral anticoagulants theophylline, phenytoin. Occasional gynaecomastia, confusion and rash
Ranitidine	150 mg twice daily or 300 mg at night	£27.00	Occasionally causes headaches and diarrhoea
Proton pump inhibitors			
Omeprazole	20–40 mg daily	£36.00– £73.00	Occasionally causes diarrhoea and headache
Lansoprazole	30 mg daily	£33.00	Occasionally causes diarrhoea and headache
Mucosal protection agents			
Sucralfate	2 g twice daily or 1 g four times daily	£14.00	Side effects include constipation and renal impairment
Misoprostol	200 μg four times daily	£20.00	Commonly causes diarrhoea

Summary of principal drugs for peptic ulceration and gastro-oesophageal reflux disease (continued)			
Drug	**Dose**	***Cost**	**Comment**
Anti-*H. pylori* drugs and combinations			
Colloidal bismuth subcitrate	2 tabs twice daily or 1 tab. four times daily for two weeks	£25.00	Care must be taken in renal impairment. Drug must be taken on an empty stomach
Metronidazole	400 mg three times daily for two weeks	£9.30	Interacts with alcohol. Can cause nausea
Amoxycillin	500 mg four times daily for two weeks	£6.00	The optimal therapy and its duration for the eradication of *H. pylori* is not known. Typical combinations include colloidal bismuth subcitrate and two antibiotics (one of which is metronizadole). More recently, small studies have shown the proton pump inhibitors and antibiotics to be effective eradication regimens
Tetracycline	500 mg four times daily for two weeks.	£3.00–£4.80	
Motility-affecting agents			
Metoclopramide	10 mg three times daily	£8.50	Extrapyramidal side effects are common in the young
Domperidone	10 mg three times daily	£6.90	May cause gynaecomastia and galactorrhoea
Cisapride	10 mg three times daily	£26.00	Occasionally causes cramp and diarrhoea
*Unless otherwise indicated, approximate cost of one month's treatment (MIMS, March 1994)			

2.2 TREATMENT OF GASTRO-OESOPHAGEAL REFLUX DISEASE

Approaches to treatment can be divided into:

* General measures
* Drug therapy
* Surgery

General measures

Symptoms can be improved by implementing several simple measures. A thorough explanation of the pathophysiology of reflux is vital, and patients should be advised to stop smoking, avoid non-steroidal anti-inflammatory (NSAID) agents when possible, avoid excessive alcohol intake and caffeine, and, if necessary, lose weight. The head of the bed should be elevated by six inches (using blocks under the bedframe and not merely relying on pillows), particularly if night-time reflux is a problem. The patient should be advised not to have a large meal shortly before going to bed.

Drug therapy

Antacids/alginates are available over the counter and are widely used by patients who self-medicate. Their effect is primarily to relieve symptoms and their use by the general practitioner can only be recommended if the patient has not already tried a regular course himself.

> **Mode of action**: Antacids neutralize the refluxed acid produced in GORD; alginates form a 'raft' over the stomach contents, thus preventing acid reflux through the gastro-oesophageal sphincter. Alginates can also offer a small acid-neutralizing effect.

Histamine-$_2$-receptor antagonists (H$_2$RAs) are appropriate in patients who have not responded to general measures and regular antacids/alginates. In many instances, treatment with H$_2$RAs relieves symptoms satisfactorily, although higher doses may be required (e.g. 300 mg ranitidine twice daily) to achieve maximum effect.

There is a vast, world-wide experience of the use of H$_2$RAs. They are remarkably well tolerated, and appear to be free from serious side effects.

The first H$_2$RA to be given a product licence was **cimetidine**, but today **ranitidine** is the most widely used. This is largely because it is better tolerated by most patients — it does not interact with the cytochrome P$_{450}$ system, which is

19

important in metabolizing a number of drugs such as warfarin, phenytoin and theophylline, and does not result in gynaecomastia, another occasional drawback of cimetidine. **Famotidine** and **nizatidine** are similar in efficacy and tolerance to ranitidine.

Mode of action: H2RAs block the histamine (H)-2 receptor of the gastric parietal cell, stimulation of which results in gastric acid secretion. Thus, their action is to inhibit secretion of gastric acid, allowing healing of peptic ulcers. ·

The **proton pump inhibitors** (omeprazole and lansoprazole) are very effective inhibitors of gastric acid secretion. The lives of many patients with severe reflux have been transformed by the use of these agents. Proton pump inhibitors are well tolerated by most people and some gastroenterologists already use them as first line therapy.

Mode of action: A proton pump inhibitor blocks H^+/K^+-ATPase, the enzyme responsible for the active secretion of hydrogen ions, and is capable of almost total suppression of both basal and stimulated gastric acid output.

Drug treatment of GORD can be initiated on a symptom-relieving basis although determination of the degree of oesophagitis is helpful in cases that do not respond to initial therapy. Oesophageal healing is an important factor in the rate of relapse of GORD. Nearly half of all patients with symptomatic GORD have no oesophagitis on endoscopy. Patients with classic heartburn do not need endoscopy in the first instance. If the symptoms are acid related they will almost certainly respond to a one month course of a proton pump inhibitor at the standard dose. If the symptoms return on cessation of treatment then endoscopy should be performed before maintenance suppression is considered.

Patients with grades 0–2 oesophagitis require the minimum level of acid suppression to control symptoms, either antacid, H2RA or proton pump inhibitor depending on response.

Endoscopic classification of oesophagitis	
Grade	
0	No oesophagitis
1	Occasional non-confluent linear red streaks
2	Confluent linear erosions
3	Ulceration
4	Complications, e.g. stricture
5	Barrett's oesophagus

Grade 3 oesophagitis (ulceration) requires treatment with a proton pump inhibitor. Healing of ulceration should be confirmed by endoscopy.

Grades 4 and 5 oesophagitis (stricture, Barrett's oesophagus) require maintenance treatment with a proton pump inhibitor.

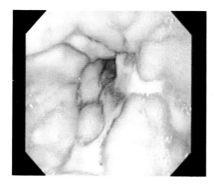 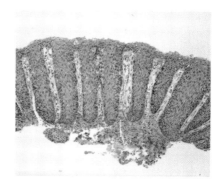

Endoscopic view of a benign oesophageal stricture and proximal oesophagitis (left). An oesophageal biopsy showing gross elongation of the papillae with a minor degree of basal cell hyperplasia and scattered inflammatory cells in the epithelium (Haematoxylin and eosin) (right). Published by permission of A Price, Northwick Park Hospital, Harrow, UK.

Endoscopy in gastro-oesophageal reflux disease

Patients who are thought to have uncomplicated reflux disease, and who respond adequately to the initial steps of the treatment strategy outlined on p22, i.e. general measures, antacids or proton pump inhibitors, do not require endoscopy. For suspected complications, particularly if dysphagia is present, endoscopy is indicated. Endoscopic grading of oesophagitis (see p20) bears little correlation to symptoms. Indeed many patients with symptomatic gastro-oesophageal reflux confirmed by pH monitoring have a completely normal endoscopy.

The presence of Barrett's oesophagus (columnar metaplasia within the oesophagus) should be confirmed by histological examination. If dysplasia is present, close follow-up will be required. Barrett's oesophagus is pre-malignant in 1–2% of cases. Although many gastroenterologists practise regular endoscopic and histological follow-up, the benefit of this approach is not proven.

If a stricture is found it should be biopsied and, if the symptoms merit, dilated.

Surgery

Approximately 5% of patients with significant GORD may require surgery. Anti-reflux surgery is very effective in relieving symptoms but complications are common and can be severe. They include: gas bloat syndrome, inability to vomit, dysphagia and recurrent GORD.

Recent laparoscopic techniques may have the advantage of minimal access and rapid recovery but the results of this surgery are not yet clear. The

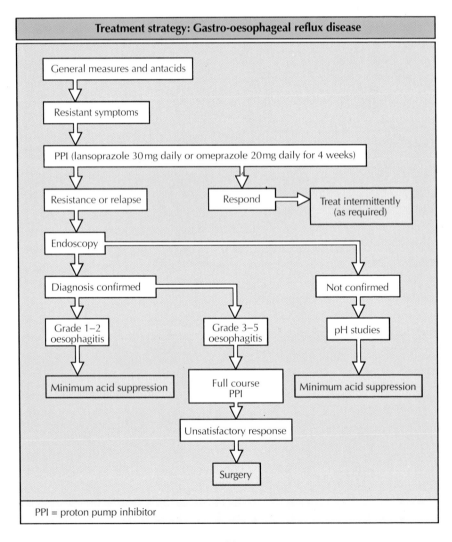

Treatment strategy: Gastro-oesophageal reflux disease

General measures and antacids

Resistant symptoms

PPI (lansoprazole 30 mg daily or omeprazole 20 mg daily for 4 weeks)

Resistance or relapse | Respond → Treat intermittently (as required)

Endoscopy

Diagnosis confirmed | Not confirmed

Grade 1–2 oesophagitis | Grade 3–5 oesophagitis | pH studies

Minimum acid suppression | Full course PPI | Minimum acid suppression

Unsatisfactory response

Surgery

PPI = proton pump inhibitor

introduction of a new operative technique is not an indication for more patients to follow that path. The initial decision should be whether the patient requires surgery at all and, second, whether laparoscopy is appropriate.

Surgery should only be considered for patients with grade 3–5 disease that is refractory to medical treatment. However, a young patient with persistent grade 1 or 2 disease may prefer surgery to the prospect of life-long mainte-nance treatment. The options should be discussed with the patient and the associated risks and benefits made clear.

2.3 TREATMENT OF DUODENAL ULCER

H$_2$RAs have been the mainstay of duodenal ulcer treatment for almost 20 years. These drugs provide good and rapid symptom relief, and are well tolerated with a low incidence of side effects. Endoscopic cure of ulceration occurs in 80% of patients after four weeks' treatment and in 90% by eight weeks with the doses previously described [2.1–2.3]. The problem with this approach is that it does not take account of the continued presence of *H. pylori* which accounts for the high rate of relapse after treatment (80% in one year). This results in the need for maintenance therapy which is both inconvenient for the patient and relatively expensive. Another caution is that long-term treatment with H$_2$RAs may relieve symptoms that would otherwise prompt further investigation and diagnosis of gastric cancer.

Proton pump inhibitors are more effective inhibitors of acid secretion than H$_2$RAs. The rate of ulcer healing (74% at two weeks; 94% at four weeks) with lansoprazole [2.4] or omeprazole [2.5] is slightly superior to that achieved with H$_2$RAs [2.6]. Rapid symptom relief occurs with treatment but, as with H$_2$RAs, the problem with recurrence after cessation of therapy also applies.

Anti-Helicobacter pylori *treatments*

Treatment of patients with duodenal ulceration has been greatly altered following the discovery of an association between duodenal ulceration and *H. pylori*. *H. pylori* cannot be said to be the only factor involved in duodenal ulcer formation because many people appear to be infected with the organism without developing an ulcer. It is clear, however, that successful eradication of infection is associated with much lower rates of relapse after ulcer healing, a fact which has rendered, by some, the eradication of *H. pylori* a primary aim in the treatment of duodenal ulcers. This approach is more attractive than maintenance with H$_2$RAs for two main reasons, namely shorter term treat-ment is both easier for the patient and less expensive.

It has been found that the rate of relapse of duodenal ulcers is reduced to around 20% in the first year if ulcer healing can be combined with anti-*H. pylori* treatment [2.7]. Because virtually all duodenal ulcers, other than those associated with NSAIDs, are associated with this infection, anti-*H. pylori* therapy can be justified in virtually all patients with duodenal ulceration.

A number of treatment regimens are effective in eradicating *H. pylori*, although, perhaps because the concept is new, comparative studies of the efficacy of different treatments are relatively few. Bismuth has anti-*H. pylori* properties, limiting its growth, but has a very low eradication rate when used alone. In combination with broad-spectrum antibiotics (**triple therapy**), bismuth produces eradication in approximately 80–90% of patients and results in a one-year relapse rate of 20% [2.8]. The acceptability of this combination is limited, however, by the relatively high incidence of side effects, particularly abdominal pain and diarrhoea. Several other combinations have been devised in order to increase the patient acceptability. The combination of the proton pump inhibitor, omeprazole, and amoxycillin (**dual therapy**) has been shown to give eradication rates of between 50–80%, while offering more rapid relief of symptoms and a higher degree of toleration [2.9]. The cost is similar to that of triple therapy but not all centres have been able to reproduce these eradication rates. Further studies are currently being carried out to find out whether other combinations are superior. Unfortunately, some strains of *H.pylori* are resistant to most conventional antibiotics and it is very difficult to eradicate the organism in such instances.

Mode of action: Triple therapy (bismuth and broad-spectrum antibiotics, usually metronidazole and tetracycline) acts as an anti-infection agent to eradicate *H. pylori*. It has no acid suppressing properties. Dual therapy (a proton pump inhibitor and broad-spectrum antibiotic) is thought to function on two fronts. The proton pump inhibitor seems to have a mild anti-*H. pylori* action in its own right but its main role is thought to be in facilitating the action of pH-sensitive antibiotics such as amoxycillin and clarithromycin.

Sucralfate

Cure rates with sucralfate are similar to those of H_2RAs but recurrence rates after treatment are lower. Whether this relates to an effect on *H. pylori* is not known.

Mode of action: Sucralfate has a cytoprotective effect; it appears to act locally by binding to the ulcer site thus preventing contact with the gastric acid. Sucralfate also promotes the local synthesis of prostaglandin E_2 which enhances the mucosal defence mechanisms.

Misoprostol

This prostaglandin analogue can be used for the treatment of duodenal ulcers although it is most commonly used in patients who have NSAID-associated gastric ulceration. It is not very effective in either symptom relief or healing of ulceration. Although it can be used to prevent the development of gastric ulcers in patients commencing treatment with NSAIDs, its use in this context should probably be restricted to patients who have previously proven peptic ulceration. It frequently causes diarrhoea, which limits tolerability. It is a potential abortifacient and should not be used in women of childbearing age.

> **Mode of action**: Prostaglandins (PGs) are potent mediators of the immune system and gastrointestinal ulceration is thought to occur as a result of low PG levels in patients receiving NSAIDS.

Treatment strategy: duodenal ulceration

There are two commonly used strategies for treating duodenal ulcers: treating the excess acid secretion or treating *H. pylori* infection.

Strategy 1: treating excess acid secretion

Use either an H_2RA (e.g. ranitidine 300 mg at night) for eight weeks or a proton pump inhibitor (e.g. lansoprazole 30 mg or omeprazole 20 mg once daily) for four weeks.

The advantages are:

- Rapid symptom relief with 90% healing rates (higher if larger doses are used for longer periods).
- Low incidence of side effects.

The disadvantages are:

- A high recurrence rate; 80% relapse by one year after cessation of treatment.

If this strategy is used then maintenance treatment with ranitidine 150 mg at night should be given in the case of frequent recurrence.

Strategy 2: Treating *H. pylori* infection

Combination therapy is essential and many treatment strategies exist but two well tried regimens are:

- Triple therapy: colloidal bismuth subcitrate (1 tablet four times daily for two weeks), tetracycline or amoxycillin (500 mg four times daily for two weeks), metronidazole (400 mg three times daily for two weeks).

- Dual therapy: lansoprazole (30 mg twice daily for four weeks) or omeprazole (40 mg once daily for four weeks) with amoxycillin (500 mg four times daily for two weeks).

The advantage of triple therapy is its greater consistent efficacy in eradicating *H. pylori* (80–90%) [2.8].

Although the relapse rate of duodenal ulceration is 80% within one year in the absence of anti-*H. pylori* intervention, certain disadvantages of this treatment exist:

- The ideal anti-*H.pylori* regimen is not known (hence the many trials using different combinations).

- Some regimens are poorly tolerated because of nausea and diarrhoea.

- Low compliance results in poor eradication [2.10]; compliance is therefore *essential* for healing.

- The organism may be resistant to metronidazole (the incidence of metronidazole-resistant organisms in the UK is currently 15%).

Dual therapy provides rapid symptom relief and ulcer healing. Claims for eradication rates are more variable (50–80%). Side effects are much fewer than for triple therapy. The problem of antibiotic resistance does not arise so frequently because metronidazole is not used.

Gastroenterologists do not agree entirely on the best strategy for treating duodenal ulcer and certainly the situation is fluid. Our current policy is to initiate treatment along the lines of strategy 2 with *dual* therapy.

2.4 TREATMENT OF RESISTANT DUODENAL ULCERATION

Several factors are associated with non-healing of duodenal ulcers. Aspects of a patient's lifestyle may delay ulcer healing; smoking and heavy alcohol intake should be discouraged. The problem of non-compliance with prescribed medication should also be considered.

In resistant ulcers (confirmed endoscopically), the *H. pylori* status should be checked and biopsies of the ulcerated lesion taken. Patients already on a proton pump inhibitor may have a false negative *H. pylori* test caused by suppression of the organism during treatment. Crohn's disease, cytomegalovirus infection and Zollinger–Ellison syndrome should also be considered.

It is our policy to use triple therapy for complicated or resistant duodenal ulcer; or maintenance treatment using a proton pump inhibitor following failure of triple therapy.

2.5 NSAID-ASSOCIATED DUODENAL ULCERATION

This condition is considered as a separate entity because ulceration can occur during treatment with NSAIDs **in the absence of *H. pylori.*** The majority of patients taking these drugs are over 60 years old, and approximately 80% of people in this group are likely to be infected with *H. pylori* [2.11]; these individuals are likely to have an especially high risk of ulceration. The role of eradicating *H. pylori* in patients with NSAID-related ulcers has not been studied. Until more is known about the possible synergism between NSAIDs and *H. pylori*, treatment should be undertaken with acid-suppressing agents.

2.6 TREATMENT OF RECURRENT DUODENAL ULCER

In practice, most duodenal ulcers, *even on the first documented diagnosis*, may be presumed to be *recurrent*. There are four groups of patients who have duodenal ulceration diagnosed at endoscopy or barium meal:

1. 'Virgin' dyspeptics who have never taken an antisecretory agent;

2. Patients who have previously taken antisecretory drugs on a symptom based diagnosis;

3. Those with known recurrent duodenal ulceration (i.e. a previously diagnosed duodenal ulcer);

4. People who have duodenal ulceration while still on treatment (i.e. a resistant duodenal ulcer).

In practice, it is very rare for the clinician to diagnose a duodenal ulcer in group 1. Most patients have a past history of dyspepsia and have taken antisecretory drugs, i.e. group 2. It is naive to suppose that this is the first time patients in this group have had a duodenal ulcer, even though it may be the first time it has been documented. Thus, most patients who have a documented ulcer have a recurrent (group 2 and 3) or resistant (group 4) duodenal ulcer. It is our policy, therefore, to treat all duodenal ulcers as recurrent as shown in the algorithm over the page. The algorithm is based on 100 patients presenting with a duodenal ulcer (presumed recurrent) and assumes at step:

a) That all duodenal ulcers may be associated with *H. pylori*. This is a safe assumption as metronidazole is not being used at this stage (obviating the problem of metronidazole resistance and aquired resistance [2.8]; b) a 50%

27

eradication rate with dual therapy (conservative estimate); c) an 80% relapse rate in people whom *H. pylori* is not successfully eradicated; d) 15% of *H. pylori* is metronidazole resistant; e) 80% eradication rate for triple therapy; f) 80% relapse rate in people who do not have successful *H. pylori* eradication.

The advantage of this regimen is that it is simple, does not require endoscopy for people who have a convincing duodenal ulcer on barium meal (and at most two endoscopies for troublesome ulcers), requires few consulations and is effective.

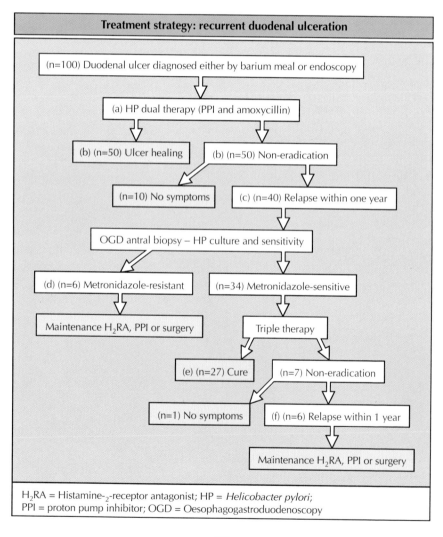

Treatment strategy: recurrent duodenal ulceration

(n=100) Duodenal ulcer diagnosed either by barium meal or endoscopy

(a) HP dual therapy (PPI and amoxycillin)

(b) (n=50) Ulcer healing → (b) (n=50) Non-eradication

(n=10) No symptoms → (c) (n=40) Relapse within one year

OGD antral biopsy – HP culture and sensitivity

(d) (n=6) Metronidazole-resistant → (n=34) Metronidazole-sensitive

Maintenance H_2RA, PPI or surgery → Triple therapy

(e) (n=27) Cure → (n=7) Non-eradication

(n=1) No symptoms → (f) (n=6) Relapse within 1 year

Maintenance H_2RA, PPI or surgery

H_2RA = Histamine-$_2$-receptor antagonist; HP = *Helicobacter pylori*;
PPI = proton pump inhibitor; OGD = Oesophagogastroduodenoscopy

Pulse therapy

Pulse therapy can be used as an alternative to maintenance treatment for the control of recurrent duodenal ulceration. Drug intervention is used on an 'as and when required' basis providing both effective symptom relief and the avoidance of unnecessary drug exposure. Symptoms should resolve after a one month course of therapy (e.g. lansoprazole 30 mg daily, omeprazole 20 mg daily or ranitidine 300 mg at night) although if drug intervention is required more than twice a year maintenance treatment is usually indicated. Pulse therapy can also be used employed on a 'weekend basis'.

2.7 SURGERY FOR DUODENAL ULCER

Surgery is clearly indicated for some complications of peptic ulcer, such as perforation, bleeding and pyloric stenosis. Its place in the management of uncomplicated ulcers is less easy to define, possibly because of the variable success rate of surgical intervention in this instance. Few people fail to respond to the potent anti-secretory agents that are available today, and in these cases the diagnosis or compliance should be questioned (see section 2.4, p26). If patients cannot comply with therapy, or if the ulcer is truly resistant, then some form of anti-ulcer operation may be indicated.

Highly selective vagotomy is the operation of choice for duodenal ulcer. It has very low morbidity and mortality. Average ulcer recurrence rates are 10–30% after five years [2.12]. Any recurrent ulcer can be treated more easily than the unwanted effects which occur following more extensive surgery. Vagotomy and drainage procedures have lower rates of ulcer recurrence, but greater post-operative morbidity. This can be very difficult to manage and many patients require additional surgery. Further details regarding the management of complications following all types of peptic ulcer surgery are given in section 3.4 (p39).

Patient advice
Patients need to be fully informed about the diagnosis, treatment, and need for investigations. The importance of stopping smoking and avoiding NSAIDs should be reinforced, and excessive use of alcohol discouraged. Many patients believe that there is a diet which helps heal ulcers, but there is no convincing evidence that this is the case. Patients should be encouraged to eat a healthy, normal diet. The importance of compliance is paramount during treatment aimed at eradicating *H. pylori*. The variations in responses in different trials suggest that the dose of drugs used is crucial; patients can be persuaded to comply with eradication regimens particularly by the relatively short periods of treatment that are now required.

General practitioner action
When a duodenal ulcer has been diagnosed, an effective ulcer healing regimen is required. There is now considerable evidence suggesting that eradication of *H. pylori* should also be attempted after the diagnosis has been made. If a satisfactory response is obtained then no further action is needed. If symptoms persist or recur shortly after a course of a proton pump inhibitor with antibiotics, an endoscopy is required to establish whether the symptoms were due to a recurrence of the duodenal ulcer. At this stage, the advice of a specialist gastroenterologist should be obtained. If the ulcer persists despite treatment, *H. pylori* status should be checked and, if positive, triple therapy instituted. If the response is inadequate or only short-lived the patient should be maintained on acid-suppressing agents, under review by the specialist; patients can be persuaded to comply with eradication regimens particularly by the relatively short periods of treatment that are now required.

2.8 TREATMENT OF GASTRIC ULCER

The treatment of gastric ulcer is more clearly defined than that of duodenal ulcer. Although evidence is mounting that *H. pylori* may be associated with gastric ulcers, eradication therapy is not usually employed at present.

Treatment options for gastric ulcer
• H2-receptor antagonists
• Proton pump inhibitors
• Misoprostol
• Sucralfate

H2-receptor antagonists

H2RAs are the traditional treatment for gastric ulcers. Treatment dosage is divided (e.g. ranitidine 150 mg twice daily), but healing and symptom relief tends to be slower than in the treatment of duodenal ulcers. After four weeks treatment at the given doses, 62% of ulcers are healed, and therefore an eight week course of H2RAs is recommended (healing rate 85%) [2.5].

Proton pump inhibitors

The rates of symptom relief and ulcer healing with proton pump inhibitors tend to be more rapid than for H2RAs, and overall success rates are higher after eight weeks treatment. If a giant gastric ulcer is diagnosed, treatment with these agents should be used in preference to H2RAs, as the healing rates are much faster. In the first instance, we suggest lansoprazole 30 mg or omeprazole 20 mg for eight weeks (healing rate 91%) [2.5]. It is our policy to treat all gastric ulcers with proton pump inhibitors.

Misoprostol

Misoprostol is less effective at healing or relieving the symptoms of gastric ulcers, even those associated with NSAIDs, than H$_2$RAs or proton pump inhibitors, and its use is limited by the high incidence of diarrhoea. In cases of NSAID-associated gastric ulceration that do not respond to acid reduction it seems sensible to try a combination of a proton pump inhibitor and misoprostol.

Sucralfate

This agent is infrequently used now, as a result of its inferior ulcer healing rate. Furthermore, the four-times daily regimen is unpopular with patients, and thus threatens compliance.

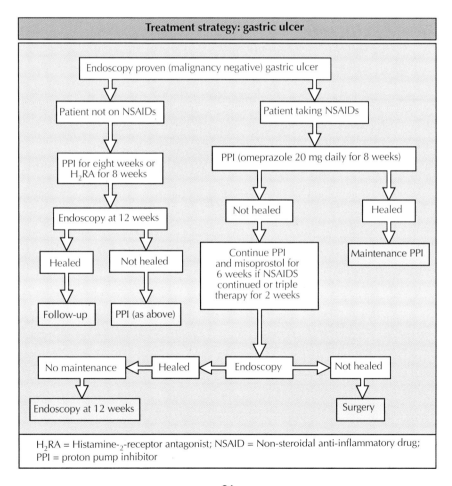

Treatment strategy: gastric ulcer

Endoscopy proven (malignancy negative) gastric ulcer

Patient not on NSAIDs

Patient taking NSAIDs

PPI for eight weeks or H$_2$RA for 8 weeks

PPI (omeprazole 20 mg daily for 8 weeks)

Endoscopy at 12 weeks

Not healed

Healed

Healed

Not healed

Continue PPI and misoprostol for 6 weeks if NSAIDS continued or triple therapy for 2 weeks

Maintenance PPI

Follow-up

PPI (as above)

No maintenance

Healed

Endoscopy

Not healed

Endoscopy at 12 weeks

Surgery

H$_2$RA = Histamine-$_2$-receptor antagonist; NSAID = Non-steroidal anti-inflammatory drug; PPI = proton pump inhibitor

General practitioner action
All patients with a suspected gastric ulcer should be referred to a gastroenterologist for investigation because of the danger of overlooking an ulcerating gastric cancer. A gastric ulcer seen on barium meal should be confirmed at endoscopy, when biopsies for histology and brushings for cytology should be taken. Following a course of ulcer healing with H2RAs or a PPI (especially if taking NSAIDs) a repeat endoscopy should be performed to confirm complete ulcer healing. Maintenance therapy is likely to be required in patients who are unable to stop taking NSAIDs, in which case a follow-up endoscopy should be done after three months maintenance treatment. The role of anti-*H. pylori* therapy is unclear in the treatment of gastric ulcers, but a trial of triple or dual therapy may be worth trying for resistant gastric ulceration. An ulcer that does not heal after a further 12 weeks treatment should be considered a medical failure and surgery must be considered. In the elderly patient who is unfit for surgery, a prolonged course of PPI and eradication therapy may be tried, although compliance is often a major problem.

Patient advice
Patients should be encouraged to stop smoking, and reduce alcohol consumption to below the advised maximum (21 units weekly for men, 14 units for women). NSAID treatment should be stopped when possible. Corticosteroids are probably not a risk factor on their own, but in combination with NSAIDs they seem to be ulcerogenic; the need for these drugs should be reviewed. No dietary restrictions are necessary, and patients need to be advised to continue treatment for the prescribed duration, and not just until symptoms are relieved.

2.9 TREATMENT OF NON-ULCER DYSPEPSIA

Antacids/alginates

These are cheap and easily available, and should be the first line of treatment in patients diagnosed as having non-ulcer dyspepsia.

H2-receptor antagonists and proton pump inhibitors

When patients fail to respond to antacids and alginates, a short trial (four weeks) of H2RAs or proton pump inhibitors can be undertaken. If the response is satisfactory, treatment can be stopped; if there is a swift recurrence of symptoms endoscopy-negative GORD should be considered as a possible diagnosis. This may be confirmed with oesophageal pH studies.

Motility drugs

Studies suggest that these agents, particularly cisapride, are of benefit in patients with non-ulcer dyspepsia, especially when bloating or volume reflux is a feature. Cisapride is relatively expensive, and it should not be prescribed long-term unless there are other specific indications.

Antispasmodics

Mebeverine, dicyclomine, and hyoscine may afford some benefit to patients with non-ulcer dyspepsia, particularly if bloating is a prominent feature and in the presence of altered bowel habit. These agents should be taken a short time before meals. Anticholinergic side effects are occasionally seen with the former two, and dicyclomine may exacerbate gastro-oesophageal reflux, although, generally speaking, these agents are well tolerated.

General practitioner action
The temptation to over-investigate patients with dyspepsia should be avoided. If symptoms continue, further reassurance may be necessary for both the patient and doctor which may then necessitate further investigation. If clinical examination, upper abdominal ultrasound, endoscopic examination and screening blood tests are normal, the patient should be strongly reassured that there is no pathological disease, and the diagnosis explained in as much detail as is required. Unless there are compounding circumstances, further investigation is unlikely to be helpful.

Patient advice
One of the most important aspects of the management of this condition is to give specific reassurance that an organic cause does not account for the symptoms while not minimising or dismissing the symptoms. A sympathetic approach and thorough explanations of the way symptoms may relate to disordered motility are often welcomed, and patients need to be reassured that the diagnosis does not lead to other diseases such as cancer. Smoking should be discouraged as this leads to overstimulation of gastric acid production, and excesses of alcohol should be discouraged. A specific diet is unlikely to relieve symptoms, but patients should avoid any foods that are consistently associated with symptoms.

2.10 TREATMENT OF GASTRITIS AND DUODENITIS

Treatment options

Symptomatic, as for non-ulcer dyspepsia (see section 2.9, p32).

Gastritis and duodenitis are endoscopic and histological diagnoses, and the belief that they can be diagnosed on the basis of specific historical clues is ill founded. A major controversy exists about whether gastritis actually causes symptoms and many studies have failed to show a correlation. It is generally accepted that duodenitis is associated with the development of duodenal ulceration, and thus a correlation with symptoms is expected. This relationship is loose, however, because many patients with duodenitis do not have symptoms. There is insufficient evidence to recommend *H. pylori* eradication therapy for these conditions [2.8].

(1)   (2)

(3)   (4)

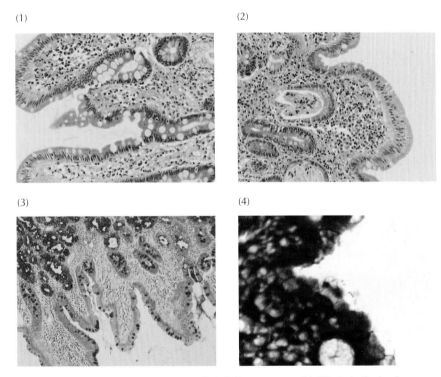

(1) Mild duodenitis characterised by a slight inflammatory cell infiltrate in the lamina propria. If this progresses to a more severe and chronic duodenitis (2), gastric-type epithelium (gastric metaplasia) may develop in the duodenal mucosa (3) (PAS stain). (4) Areas of gastric metaplasia in duodenal mucosa can be colonised by *H. pylori* (Gimenez stain), and this can subsequently lead to frank duodenal ulcer.
Published by permission of MJ Walker, St Mary's Hospital, London, UK.

3 Appendices

3.1 *HELICOBACTER PYLORI*

Spiral organisms have been noted in the stomach for the last 100 years but it was Marshall and Warren [3.1–3.3] who observed and cultured small S-shaped bacilli from biopsy material of patients with gastritis and introduced the modern era of *Campylobacter pylori*, now named *Helicobacter pylori*.

H. pylori thrives in the mucus layer of the gastric antrum, both on the surface and in the crypts. *H. pylori* is not found in the duodenal mucosa but if gastric metaplasia has occurred in the duodenum (see p34) it may be found in the gastric-type metaplastic mucosa. *H. pylori* produces an enzyme called urease which creates a local alkaline environment in the surrounding mucus.

Epidemiology
The prevalence of *H. pylori* increases with age and decreasing socio-economic status. In developed countries the prevalence increases from 20% in 20 year old individuals to 50% in 50 year old individuals. In the Third World, *H. pylori* is ubiquitous with up to 75% of 20 year olds affected and up to 98% of the population aged 50 years.

Detection of **H. pylori**

- Histology (endoscopic biopsy)

- Culture (endoscopic biopsy)

- Biopsy urease (CLO) test

- $^{13/14}$C-urea breath test

- Serum IgA antibody to *H. pylori*

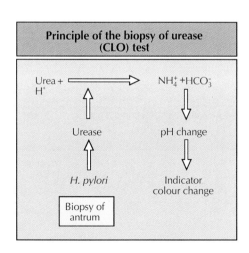

Principle of the biopsy of urease (CLO) test

$$Urea + H^+ \Longrightarrow NH_4^+ + HCO_3^-$$

Urease → pH change

H. pylori → Indicator colour change

Biopsy of antrum

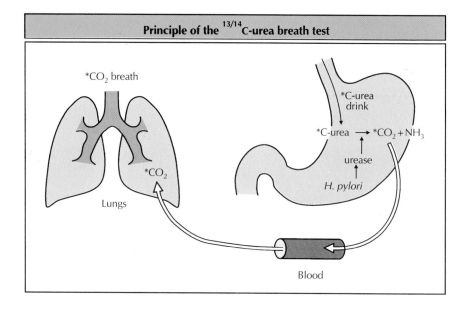

Principle of the $^{13/14}$C-urea breath test

*CO$_2$ breath

*C-urea drink

*C-urea ⟶ *CO$_2$+NH$_3$

urease

H. pylori

*CO$_2$

Lungs

Blood

Pathogenicity

Not everyone with *H. pylori* has disease. It is a heterogenous organism and some strains are more pathogenic. Experimental ingestion, however, has resulted in acute gastritis [3.4,3.5], therefore fulfilling Koch's postulates for a causal relationship.

Treatment

H. pylori is strongly associated with duodenal ulcer relapse which has added to the maxim 'No acid, no ulcer', 'No *H. pylori*, no ulcer'. If *H. pylori* is eradicated very few duodenal ulcers relapse. Eradicating *H. pylori* cures the disease [3.6]. Many gastroenterologists recommend *H. pylori* eradication for duodenal ulcer disease (this is our policy).

Disease associations	
Disease	**Approximate incidence**
Duodenal ulcer	95%
Antral gastritis	90%
Gastric ulcer	75%
Non-ulcer dyspepsia	40–60%
Asymptomatic population	20–50%
Patients on NSAIDS with a duodenal ulcer have a lower prevalence of infection (75%), as do those with a perforated duodenal ulcer	

H. pylori eradication may become common practice for gastric ulceration but it is not yet generally accepted (it is not our policy). The role of *H. pylori* eradication in the epidemiology of gastric cancer needs to be addressed. At present, widespread *H. pylori* eradication is not indicated.

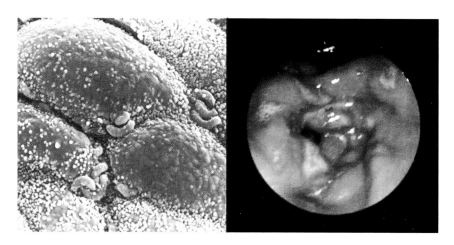

Helicobacter pylori in the gastric antrum (left); scanning EM x 60,000. Severe erosive/ulcerative inflammation in the antrum (right), with acute histological *H. pylori*-associated inflammation in a young patient with sudden severe dyspepsia. Published by permission of MJ Walker, St Mary's Hospital, London, UK and GNJ Tytgat, Academic Medical Centre, Amsterdam, The Netherlands.

3.2 GASTRO-OESOPHAGEAL REFLUX DISEASE

A degree of reflux of gastric contents is demonstrable in healthy individuals. Patients with symptomatic (pathological) reflux tend to have longer periods of reflux due to impaired oesophageal clearance of refluxate, or demonstrate excessive oesophageal sensitivity to the presence of acid and/or food. Reflux is commonly associated with a hiatus hernia, but other causes of increased reflux include:

• Pregnancy or obesity

• Fat, chocolate or coffee ingestion

• Smoking

• Anticholinergic drugs

• Systemic sclerosis

Oesophagitis is the inflammation that occurs as a result of refluxed gastric contents: it can be diagnosed endoscopically or histologically. Although the presence of oesophagitis infers that reflux is occurring, its absence does not exclude the possibility of significant reflux. Less than half of all patients with significant and symptomatic reflux do not have endoscopic oesophagitis.

Timing of reflux

Reflux most typically occurs at night when the patient lies flat (see figure below), but other patterns of reflux are recognised, particularly after meals.

Refluxate

Acid is the most easily identifiable component of the refluxate, but other components of the gastric contents probably have important roles in the causation of symptoms. These include pepsin, food and bile.

Pathophysiology

Gastro-oesophageal reflux is often associated with impaired lower oesophageal sphincter tone. It may cause symptoms by the following mechanisms:

- Erosion and ulceration leading to inflammation (although this is probably not the major mechanism as there is a poor correlation between symptoms and degree of inflammation).

- The production of reflux spasm in the oesophagus.

- Nocturnal bronchospasm (which may be preceded by reflux).

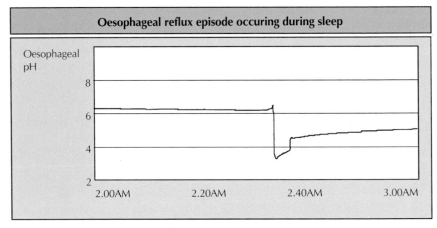

Reflux episode occurring during sleep while oesophageal pH monitoring is taking place. Note the long period before the intraoesophageal pH falls to 4.

3.3 BARRETT'S OESOPHAGUS

Barrett's oesophagus is defined as the presence of columnar metaplasia in the oesophagus, usually beginning at the oesophagogastric junction and extending proximally for at least 3 cm. It is thought to occur as a result of gastro-oesophageal reflux and can lead to complications such as ulceration, stricturing, and dysplasia and carcinoma.

It is thought that dysplastic changes in Barrett's oesophagus may herald frank carcinoma. Therefore, regular endoscopic surveillance of patients with this disorder has been advocated. The benefits of intensive screening are as yet unproven. Our practice is to screen with endoscopic biopsies every two years. A more aggressive approach might be adopted in young patients with extensive metaplasia, and in smokers.

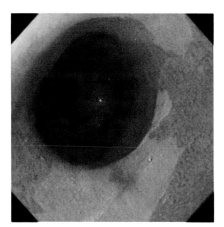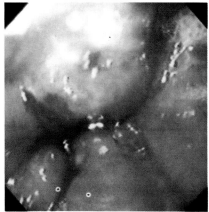

Endoscopic view of Barrett's oesophagus; this is pre-malignant in 1–2% of cases. The light pink mucosa is normal squamous oesophageal epithelium. The dark pink area is metaplastic (Barrett's) columnar epithelium. The oesophagosquamous junction is 7 cm above the gastro-oesophageal junction seen in the distance (left). Endoscopic view of an adenocarcinoma in a Barrett's oesophagus (right).

3.4 MANAGEMENT OF POST-OPERATIVE COMPLICATIONS

Most patients who have surgery for peptic ulcer, gallstones, or gastro-oesophageal reflux will have their symptoms improved. There is, however, a sizeable portion of patients whose symptoms are not relieved by surgery, and management of this group can be extremely difficult. Published figures on rates of complication and symptom recurrence are prone to bias, and almost certainly under estimate the prevalence of these problems.

Immediate post-operative complications will generally be dealt with by the surgeons who performed the operation, and their management is beyond the scope of this text. It is assumed that the reader is more likely to be presented with a patient who has a delayed complication of, or a poor result from, surgery. Some attempt at clarification of the common post-operative problems, and their management, follows.

Is the operation really necessary and is it appropriate?

This may seem like an unnecessary question because all surgeons presumably perform surgery in the belief that the operation is necessary, in the expectation of helping the patient. However, there is good evidence that some operations are performed largely because the operation is available; for example, it is known that the number of cholecystectomies performed varies from region to region, and that this variation correlates very closely with the number of surgeons who are interested in this work.

The symptom overlap in dyspeptic conditions has been discussed, and a thorough assessment and series of investigations are needed before surgery is undertaken. It should be remembered that fatty food intolerance is no more frequent in patients with gallstones than in those without. Before we advise patients to undergo an operation, we should be clear that the operation is clinically indicated. The most sure way of avoiding post-operative complications is not to perform the operation in the first instance! It is also expedient to avoid certain types of surgery in particular cases, for example, the risk of gastric cancer is increased following gastric resection and so, when possible, this type of surgery should be avoided in young patients.

Specific post-operative problems

Dysphagia and **gas-bloat syndrome** are common in the immediate post-operative period, occurring in up to 50% of patients, as a result of oedema and haematoma. These symptoms soon settle and patients should be reassured. Symptoms may persist in a minority (2%) of patients, and endoscopic dilation or a conversion of a Nissen fundoplication to a floppier repair is occasionally necessary. Gas-bloat syndrome needs to be distinguished from inadvertent vagotomy, which results in **gastroparesis**, and is usually associated with vomiting. A succussion splash may be evident. Recurrent **gastro-oesophageal reflux** should be treated medically in the first instance (see p19).

Post operative syndromes of anti-reflux surgery
• Dysphagia
• Gas-bloat syndrome (bloating due to inability to belch)
• Gastric stasis
• Recurrent gastro-oesophageal reflux

Syndromes that occur after ulcer surgery or other gastric surgery

Several post-operative syndromes are recognised following gastric surgery. These will be considered separately but can co-exist.

Diarrhoea

Diarrhoea can be quite debilitating, and particularly so in patients who have had both gastric surgery and cholecystectomy. It is likely to be multifactorial and result from:

- Loss of pyloric hold-up
- Effect of vagotomy on intestinal tone
- Loss of co-ordination between pancreatic juice, bile and food
- Reduced gastric acid production causing malabsorption

It is important to exclude other diseases such as colonic cancer and colitis. The following may also be of benefit in some patients but should only be continued if there is a definite subjective improvement:

- Broad-spectrum antibiotics
- Exclusion of milk products from diet
- Codeine phosphate 15–30 mg four hourly
- Diphenoxylate 5 mg six hourly
- Octreotide

Corrective surgery or insertion of a 'reverse loop' may occasionally be necessary if symptoms persist.

Small stomach syndrome

Part of the stomach's function is to act as a capacitance vessel for food. It should not, therefore, be surprising if the stomach feels full after a small meal when some of it has been removed. Patients should be reassured that adaptation occurs.

Dumping (early)

Early dumping is due to hypovolaemia, which occurs after the rapid arrival of food in the small intestine (which acts as an osmotic load). Symptoms typically occur within 15 minutes of a meal, and include weakness, dizziness and fainting. Distension, colic and diarrhoea are also common.

Post-operative syndromes of gastric surgery
• Diarrhoea
• Small stomach syndrome
• Dumping syndrome (early and late)
• Bile reflux

Dumping (late)

Late dumping occurs as a result of reflex hyperinsulinaemia, which leads to hypoglycaemia, following the arrival and subsequent absorption of a large sugar and fatty acid load at the small intestine. Hunger, shakiness, tachycardia and sweating are the main symptoms.

Dumping occurs in approximately 30% of patients immediately following gastric surgery. Patients should be reassured that adaptation occurs but that this may take up to 12 months in some instances. Small, frequent, dry meals should be advised. In severe and persistent cases, a reconstruction may be necessary.

Bile reflux

This can occur in any operation where the pylorus has been resected or by-passed but particularly after a polya partial gastrectomy. Typically, the patient will complain bitterly about the appearance of bile in the mouth, with or without heartburn. Acid suppressing agents are of little benefit, and alginates and antacids do not appear to help. Patients will occasionally respond to motility-affecting drugs, but the symptoms are often so severe that further surgery is necessary.

Post-cholecystectomy syndrome

This is a common problem and the similarity between the syndrome and the symptoms for which the operation was performed are frequently striking. Patients complain of biliary type pain, frequently with some degree of scar tenderness. There is often nausea but no vomiting. The pain typically occurs in frequent exacerbations, and there may be associated diarrhoea (see opposite).

Its aetiology is disputed, but elevated bile duct pressure and bile duct dyskinesia have been demonstrated in a number of cases, although normal controls are difficult to study.

Retained bile duct calculi should be excluded by measuring liver function tests and performing a bile duct ultrasound.

Treatment

- Nifedipine

- Mebeverine

- Endoscopic sphincterotomy (its role is disputed)

Post-cholecystectomy diarrhoea

When the gall bladder is removed, bile drips slowly into the duodenum, irrespective of the presence of food. This can lead to the following:

- Bile salts passing into the colon, unbuffered by food, where they become irritant and result in cholorrhoeic diarrhoea.

or rarely

- Bile salt defiency, as a result of loss of the bile salt pool, which can result in steatorrhoea.

Treatment

- Cholorrhoeic diarrhoea – cholestyramine 4 g up to six times daily

- Bile salt deficiency – this may be helped by altering the diet to reduce fat intake.

3.5 PEPTIC ULCER HAEMORRHAGE

Bleeding peptic ulcers may present with classical symtoms of haematemesis and malaena. Care should be taken to look for the atypical presentation, e.g. lethargy, syncope, angina, precipitated by hypovolaemia. Patients with sus-pected peptic ulcer haemorrhage should be admitted to hospital urgently. The patient should be examined for pallor and blood pressure recorded. Once in hospital, haemoglobin levels will be checked, together with urea and elec-trolytes and central venous pressure monitored when appropriate. Endoscopy will be performed at the first available opportunity after the patient has been adequately resuscitated.

Identifying the high risk group

Specific risk factors associated with a high risk of mortality following upper gastrointestinal haemorrhage are:

- Age over 65 years

- Anticoagulant or NSAID therapy

- Concomitant cardiorespiratory disease

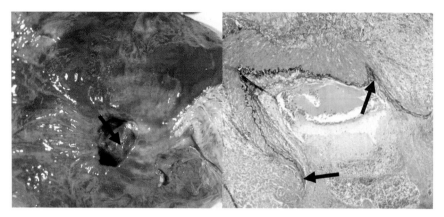

Benign peptic ulcer on the lesser curvature of the stomach (left); the arrow indicates the presence of a ruptured artery in the base of the ulcer, which resulted in haemorrhage. Small artery in the base of the gastric ulcer (right) from the *post mortem* specimen shown on the left; staining shows rupture of the artery at the points arrowed. Published by permission of MJ Walker, St Mary's Hospital, London, UK.

Likelihood of recurrent bleeding

The following are associated with an increased risk of recurrent or continued bleeding from a peptic ulcer which necessitates surgical intervention:

- Anticoagulants/coagulopathy;

- Endoscopic stigmata; visible vessel within ulcer (endoscopic intervention is especially helpful in this instance);

- Red spots within an ulcer (less strongly associated with rebleeding).

Immediate treatment

- Resuscitation with intravenous fluids and/or blood.

- Close monitoring, if possible within a designated gastrointestinal bleeding unit or high dependency area.

- Endoscopic treatment will depend on the cause of the bleeding.

Bleeding varices will be treated with injection therapy or banding. A bleeding peptic ulcer with stigmata suggests that rebleeding is likely and will require injection sclerotherapy or diathermy/LASER treatment.

When patients rebleed from a peptic ulcer despite endoscopic treatment, surgery is recommended, except in exceptional cases which should be evaluated by the gastroenterologist and surgeon. When bleeding from oesophageal varices recurs after sclerotherapy, a period of tamponade, using a Sengstaken tube, is required; specific precautions to prevent hepatic encephalopathy are usually necessary.

Long-term treatment

Patients who have suffered major bleeding, requiring transfusion, from a peptic ulcer should be monitored endoscopically to check that satisfactory healing has occurred. Patients with a gastric ulcer should probably receive maintenance therapy to prevent recurrence, people with a duodenal ulcer should receive *H. pylori* eradication with triple therapy (see p25). Eradication should be confirmed (see section 3.1) and, if failed, maintenance treatment commenced (see p26).

3.6 GASTRIC ULCERATION

Prepyloric gastric ulcers are associated with a high gastric acid production. They have many other epidemiological similarities to duodenal ulcers. Most patients with gastric ulcers in the gastric antrum or corpus have a low gastric acid output, and other factors may be important in the pathogenesis of the ulceration. These include:

- Altered mucus production
- Duodenogastric reflux of bile
- Mucosal ischaemia (?prostaglandin mediated)
- *H. pylori* infection

3.7 DUODENAL ULCERATION

People with duodenal ulcer disease have a higher parietal cell mass than healthy individuals, and a greater acid output. Approximately 15% of the population will suffer from a duodenal ulcer at some time, and there is a fourfold greater incidence in men than in women. Factors which are thought to play a role in the development of ulceration include the following.

Genetic

There is a strong family association. This may be linked to the inheritance of non-secretion of blood group antigens into the gastric secretions, or to the inheritance of various genes which encode for pepsin.

Environmental

- Smoking

- Aspirin and NSAIDs

- Corticosteroids (probably do not cause ulceration but are associated with an increased risk in patients also taking NSAIDs)

- *H. pylori* (see p35)

- Geography (more frequent in Scotland and north of England)

- Loose correlation with low socio-economic class

- Diet, alcohol and psychological factors, including stress, have not been conclusively shown to have any effect on the pathogenesis of this disease

Disease associations

- Hyperparathyriodism/hypercalcaemia

- Renal failure

- Zollinger–Ellison syndrome

3.8 ZOLLINGER–ELLISON SYNDROME

This is a rare endocrine tumour that produces gastrin. In common with many other endocrine tumours, additional hormones may be synthesized which can be detected either in the blood or the resected tumour.

Pancreatic gastrinomas can be associated with other endocrine tumours, particularly parathyroid adenoma and pituitary adenoma, as part of the multiple endocrine neoplasia spectrum of disease.

Features

Recurrent ulceration, particularly if associated with the following, should alert the doctor to the possibility of this diagnosis:

- Large and multiple ulcers which respond poorly to treatment

- Ulcers in the second, or more distal, part of the duodenum

- Complications (haemorrhage or perforation)

- Diarrhoea

- Hypercalcaemia

- Recurrent ulceration following peptic ulcer surgery

Diagnosis

- Raised (fasting) serum gastrin and high basal acid output (>15 mmol/h).
- Serum gastrin increases markedly in reponse to i.v. secretin (2 u/kg).

Treatment

- Proton pump inhibitors in high doses (e.g. omeprazole 100 mg daily)
- Surgery

Gastrinomas are frequently multiple and are commonly malignant. In younger patients, an attempt at curative excision should be made in specialized centres. The tumours typically occur in the head of the pancreas and the duodenal wall, and a combination of CAT scanning, angiography, and laparotomy with on-table enteroscopy and duodenal transillumination have been described as the optimal method for their complete removal.

3.9 MODE OF ACTION OF DRUGS USED IN THE TREATMENT OF DYSPEPSIA

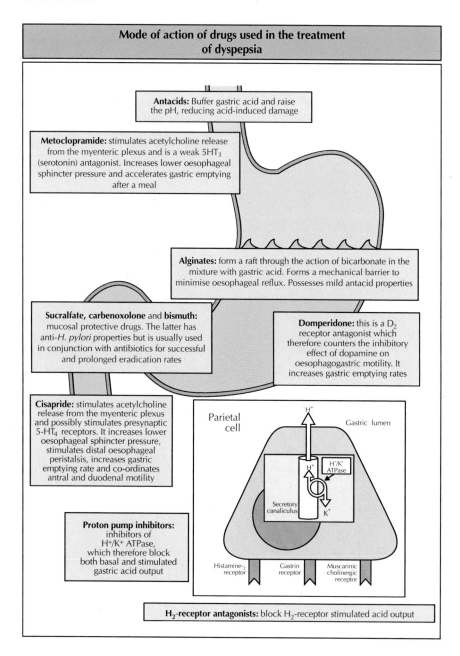

Mode of action of drugs used in the treatment of dyspepsia

Antacids: Buffer gastric acid and raise the pH, reducing acid-induced damage

Metoclopramide: stimulates acetylcholine release from the myenteric plexus and is a weak 5HT$_3$ (serotonin) antagonist. Increases lower oesophageal sphincter pressure and accelerates gastric emptying after a meal

Alginates: form a raft through the action of bicarbonate in the mixture with gastric acid. Forms a mechanical barrier to minimise oesophageal reflux. Possesses mild antacid properties

Sucralfate, carbenoxolone and **bismuth:** mucosal protective drugs. The latter has anti-*H. pylori* properties but is usually used in conjunction with antibiotics for successful and prolonged eradication rates

Domperidone: this is a D$_2$ receptor antagonist which therefore counters the inhibitory effect of dopamine on oesophagogastric motility. It increases gastric emptying rates

Cisapride: stimulates acetylcholine release from the myenteric plexus and possibly stimulates presynaptic 5-HT$_4$ receptors. It increases lower oesophageal sphincter pressure, stimulates distal oesophageal peristalsis, increases gastric emptying rate and co-ordinates antral and duodenal motility

Parietal cell

Gastric lumen

H^+

H^+

H^+/K^+ ATPase

Secretory canaliculus

K^+

Proton pump inhibitors: inhibitors of H+/K+ ATPase, which therefore block both basal and stimulated gastric acid output

Histamine-$_2$ receptor

Gastrin receptor

Muscarinic cholinergic receptor

H$_2$-receptor antagonists: block H$_2$-receptor stimulated acid output

References

Part 1

1.1 Davenport PM, Morgan AG, Darnborough A, *et al.*: **Can preliminary screening of dyspeptic patients allow more effective use of investigational techniques?** *BMJ* 1985, **290**:217–220.

1.2 Crean GP, Card WI, Beattie AD, *et al.*: **Ulcer-like dyspepsia.** *Scand J Gastroenterol* 1982, **17**(Suppl 79):9–15.

Part 2

2.1 Nwokolo CU, Smith JTL, Gavey C, *et al.*: **Tolerance during 29 days of conventional dosing with cimetidine, nizatidine, famotidine or ranitidine** *Aliment Pharmacol Ther* 1990, **4**(suppl 1):29–45.

2.2 Page MC, Lacey LA, Mills JG, *et al.*: **Can higher doses of an H$_2$ receptor antagonist accelerate duodenal ulcer healing?** *Aliment Pharmacol Ther* 1989, **3**:425–433.

2.3 McFarland RJ, Bateson MC, Green JRB, *et al.*: **Omeprazole provides quicker symptom relief and duodenal ulcer healing than ranitidine**. *Gastroenterology* 1990, **98**:278–283.

2.4 Londong W: **Dose related healing of duodenal ulcer with the proton pump inhibitor lansoprazole.** *Aliment Pharmacol Ther 1991*, **5**:245–254.

2.5 Blum AL: **Treatment of acid-related disorders with gastric acid inhibitors: the state of the art.** *Digestion* 1990, **41**(suppl 1):3–10.

2.6 Pounder RE, Nwokolo CU: **Duodenal ulceration.** In *Recent Advances In Gastroenterology, Number 8*, edited by Pounder RE. Edinburgh: Churchill Livingstone 1990, pp 117–131.

2.7 Marshall B, Goodwin CS, Warren JR, *et al.*: **Prospective double-blind trial of duodenal ulcer relapse after eradication of *Campylobacter pylori*.** *Lancet* 1988, **2**:1437–1442.

2.8 Tytgat GNJ, Axon ATR, Dixon MF, *et al.*: **Helicobacter pylori: causal agent in peptic ulcer disease?** In *Working Party Report of the World Congress of Gastroenterology*. Sydney: Blackwell Scientific Publications 1990, pp 36–45.

2.9 Labenz J, Gyenes E, Rühl GH, *et al.*: **Amoxycillin plus omeprazole versus triple therapy for eradication of *Helicobacter pylori* in duodenal ulcer disease: a prospective, randomized and controlled study.** *Gut* 1993, **34**:1167–1170.

2.10 Graham DY, Lew GM, Malaty HM, *et al.*: **Factors influencing the eradication of *Helicobacter pylori* with triple therapy**. *Gastroenterology* 1992, **102**:493–496.

2.11 Graham DY, Klein PD, Opekun AR, *et al.*: **Effect of age on the frequency of active Campylobacter pylori infection diagnosed by the [^{13}C] urea breath test in normal subjects and patients with peptic ulcer disease.** *J Infect Dis* 1988, **157**:777–780.

2.12 Carter DC. **Surgical management of peptic ulcer.** In *Diseases of the Gut and Pancreas*, 2nd edn, edited by Misiewicz JJ, Pounder RE, Venables CW. Oxford: Blackwell Scientific Publications 1994, pp 291–301.

Part 3

3.1 Warren JR, Marshall BJ: **Unidentified curved bacilli on gastric epithelium in active chronic gastritis.** *Lancet* 1983, **i**:1273–1275.

3.2 Marshall BJ, Warren JR: **Unidentified curved bacilli in the stomach of patients with gastritis and peptic ulceration.** *Lancet* 1984, **i**:1311–1315.

3.3 Rollason TP, Stone J, Rhodes JM: **Spiral organisms in endoscopic biopsies of the human stomach.** *J Clin Pathol* 1984, **37**:23–26.

3.4 Marshall BJ, Armstrong JA, McGechie DB, *et al.*: **Attempt to fulfil Koch's postulates for pyloric *Campylobacter*.** *Med J Aust* 1985, **142**:436–439.

3.5 Morris A, Nicholson G: **Ingestion of *Campylobacter pyloridis* causes gastritis and raised fasting pH.** *Am J Gastroenterol* 1987, **82**:192–199.

3.6 Rauws EAJ, Tytgat GNJ: **Cure of duodenal ulcer associated with eradication of *Helicobacter pylori*.** *Lancet* 1990, **335**:1233–1235.

Further reading

1. Festen HPM: **Can the natural history of duodenal ulcer disease be altered?** *Eur J Gastro Hepatol* 1993, **5**:307–309.

2. Taha AS, Russell RI: **Helicobacter pylori and non-steroidal anti-inflammatory drugs: uncomfortable partners in peptic ulcer disease.** *Gut* 1993, **34**:580–583.

3. Brown C, Rees WDW: **Dyspepsia in general practice.** *BMJ* 1990, **300**:829–830.

4. McColl KEL, Fullarton GM. **Duodenal ulcer pain: the role of acid and inflammation.** *Gut* 1993, **34**:1300–1302.

5. Langman MJS, Brooks P, Hawkey CJ, *et al.*: **Working party report to the World Congress of Gastroenterology, Sydney, 1990. Non-steroidal anti-inflammatory drug associated ulcer: epidemiology, causation and treatment.** *J Gastro Hepatol* 1991, **6**:442–449.

6. Moss S, Calam J: *Helicobacter pylori* **and peptic ulcers: the present position.** *Gut* 1992, **33**:289–292.

7. Axon AR: **Duodenal ulcer: the villain unmasked?** *BMJ* 1991, **302**:919–921.

8. Feldman M, Burton ME: **Histamine$_2$-receptor antagonists. Standard therapy for acid-peptic diseases (first of two parts).** *N Engl J Med* 1990, **323**: 1672– 1680.

9. Feldman M, Burton ME. **Histamine$_2$-receptor antagonists. Standard therapy for acid-peptic diseases (second of two parts).** *N Engl J Med* 1990, **323**: 1749–1755.

10. The Eurogast Study Group: **An international association between** *Helicobacter pylori* **infection and gastric cancer.** *Lancet* 1993, **341**:1359–1362.

11. Colin-Jones DG, Langman MJS, Lawson DH, *et al.*: **Postmarketing surveillance of the safety of cimetidine: 10 year mortality report.** *Gut* 1992, **33**:1280–1284.

12. Alexander-Williams J: **A requiem for vagotomy.** *BMJ* 1991, **302**:547–548.

13. Loft DE. **Postoperative problems**. In *Clinical gastroenterology,* edited by Turnberg LA. Oxford: Blackwell Scientific Publications 1989, pp 404–434.

14. Fennerty MB, Sampliner E, Garewal HS: **Review article: Barrett's oesophagus — cancer risk, biology and therapeutic management**. *Aliment Pharmacol Ther* 1993, **7**:339–345.

15. Walt RP: **Upper gastrointestinal bleeding.** In *Recent Advances In Gastroenterology, Number 8,* edited by Pounder RE. Edinburgh: Churchill Livingstone 1990, pp 101–116.

16. Smith JTL, Gavey C, Nwokolo CU, *et al.*: **Tolerance during 8 days of high-dose H$_2$-blockade: placebo controlled studies of 24 hour acidity and gastrin.** *Aliment Pharmacol Ther* 1990, **4**(suppl 1):47–63.

17. Nwokolo CU, Mistry P, Pounder RE: **The absorption of bismuth and salicylate from oral doses of pepto-bismol (bismuth salicylate).** *Aliment Pharmacol Ther* 1990, **4**:163–169.

18. Jones R, Lydeard S: **Dyspepsia in the community: a follow up study.** *Br J Clin Pract* 1992, **46**:95–97.

19. Loft DE. **Problems after surgery.** *Med Int* 1986, **17**:1102–1195.

20. Mohammed R, Hearns JB, Crean GP: **Gastric acid secretion in children with duodenal ulceration.** *Scan J Gastroenterol* 1982, **17**:289–292.

21. Shorvon PJ, Loft DE. **Radiology and endoscopy of the stomach and duodenum.** In *Diseases of the Gut and Pancreas*, 2nd edn, edited by Misiewicz JJ, Pounder RE, Venables CW. Oxford: Blackwell Scientific Publications 1994, pp187–207.

Index